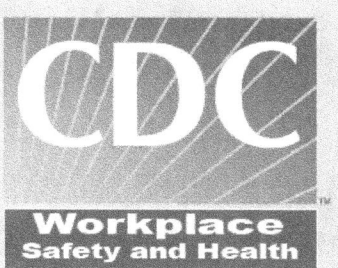

Environmental and Biological Assessment of Environmental Tobacco Smoke Exposure Among Casino Dealers

Chandran Achutan, PhD
Christine West, RN, MSN, MPH
Charles Mueller, MS
Yvonne Boudreau, MD, MSPH
Kenneth Mead, PhD, PE

Health Hazard Evaluation Report
HETA 2005-0076; 2005-0201-3080
Bally's, Paris, and Caesars Palace Casinos
Las Vegas, Nevada
May 2009

DEPARTMENT OF HEALTH AND HUMAN SERVICES
Centers for Disease Control and Prevention

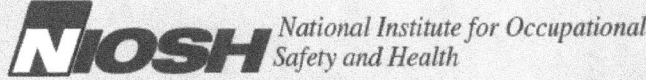
National Institute for Occupational
Safety and Health

The employer shall post a copy of this report for a period of 30 calendar days at or near the workplace(s) of affected employees. The employer shall take steps to insure that the posted determinations are not altered, defaced, or covered by other material during such period. [37 FR 23640, November 7, 1972, as amended at 45 FR 2653, January 14, 1980].

CONTENTS

ABBREVIATIONS

4-VP	4-vinyl pyridine
ACGIH®	American Conference of Governmental Industrial Hygienists
ACTLD	Acetaldehyde
ALD	Aldehyde
ANSI	American National Standards Institute
API	Atmospheric-pressure ionization
ASHRAE	American Society of Heating, Refrigerating and Air-Conditioning Engineers
ASTM	American Society for Testing and Materials
cfm	Cubic feet per minute
CO	Carbon monoxide
CO_2	Carbon dioxide
COT	Cotinine
°F	Degrees Fahrenheit
EPA	Environmental Protection Agency
ETS	Environmental tobacco smoke
FLD	Formaldehyde
fpm	Feet per minute
GC	Gas chromatography
GM	Geometric mean
HHE	Health hazard evaluation
HPLC	High performance liquid chromatography
HVAC	Heating, ventilation, and air conditioning
IEQ	Indoor environmental quality
LOD	Limit of detection
LOQ	Limit of quantitation
Lpm	Liters per minute
MDC	Minimum detectable concentration
MERV	Minimum efficiency reporting value
min	Minute(s)
mg/m^3	Milligrams per cubic meter
mL	Milliliter
mm	Millimeter
MS	Mass spectrometry
n	Sample size
ng	Nanogram

ABBREVIATIONS
(CONTINUED)

NIC	Nicotine
NIOSH	National Institute for Occupational Safety and Health
nmol/mgcr	Nanomoles per milligrams of creatinine
NNAL	4-(Methylnitrosamino)-1-(3-pyridyl)-1-butanol
NNK	4-(Methylnitrosamino)-1-(3-pyridyl)-1-butanone
NP	Nonpoker
NRT	Nicotine replacement therapy
OEL	Occupational exposure limit
OSHA	Occupational Safety and Health Administration
OVS	OSHA versatile sampler
PAH	Polynuclear aromatic hydrocarbon
PBZ	Personal breathing zone
PEL	Permissible exposure limit
PFTE	Polytetrafluoroethylene
pg	Picogram
pmol/mgcr	Picomoles per milligrams of creatinine
ppb	Parts per billion
ppm	Parts per million
r	Pearson's correlation coefficient
REL	Recommended exposure limit
RH	Relative humidity
RSP	Respirable suspended particulates
SOL	Solanesol
STEL	Short-term exposure limit
THC	Total hydrocarbon (as toluene)
TLV®	Threshold limit value
TOL	Toluene
TWA	Time-weighted average
UV	Ultraviolet
VOC	Volatile organic compound
μL	Microliter
μg/m^3	Micrograms per cubic meter
μm	Micrometer
WEEL	Workplace environmental exposure limit

National Institute for Occupational Safety and Health (NIOSH) investigators evaluated environmental tobacco smoke (ETS) exposure at Bally's, Paris, and Caesars Palace casinos in Las Vegas, Nevada, at the request of casino employees. They measured exposures and surveyed employees about health symptoms. They found evidence of workplace exposure to a tobacco-specific carcinogen among non-poker casino dealers. Based on the known link between ETS and health effects, NIOSH investigators recommend establishing casino-wide no smoking policies and developing smoking cessation programs for casino employees.

What NIOSH Did

- We talked to nonpoker (NP) casino dealers about symptoms that may have been related to ETS exposure.
- We took personal breathing zone and area air samples to measure ETS.
- We took urine samples to see if components of ETS were absorbed into NP casino dealers' bodies.
- We surveyed NP casino dealers and casino office staff about their work, medical problems, and symptoms.

What NIOSH Found

- NP casino dealers reported having respiratory symptoms. They thought these symptoms were related to ETS.
- We found ETS components in the air. These components include nicotine, 4-vinyl pyridine, respirable dust, solanesol, benzene, toluene, p-dichloromethane, naphthalene, formaldehyde, and acetaldehyde.
- We found increased urinary levels of one ETS component during the work shift. This finding shows that these components were absorbed in NP casino dealers' bodies.
- More NP casino reported respiratory symptoms than administrative and engineering employees, but the differences between the groups were not statistically significant.

What Casino Managers Can Do

- Ban smoking in the casinos.
- Offer smoking cessation classes for employees.
- Make sure that ventilation systems are working properly.
- Form health and safety committees with employees and managers. These committees should meet regularly to address employee health concerns.

What Casino Employees Can Do

- Stop smoking.
- See a doctor for any health concerns or symptoms.
- Take part in casino health and safety committees.

SUMMARY

Evidence of workplace exposure to ETS was demonstrated by a measurable increase of a biological marker (NNAL), a known lung carcinogen, over a work shift in NP casino dealers. NP casino dealers reported higher prevalence of respiratory symptoms than administrative and engineering workers unexposed to ETS at work, but these differences were not statistically significant. The casinos should institute casino-wide no smoking policies and develop smoking cessation programs for their employees.

Between January and April 2005, NIOSH received confidential requests for HHEs from NP casino dealers at Bally's, Paris, and Caesars Palace casinos in Las Vegas, Nevada. These casino dealers were concerned that exposure to ETS in their workplace was causing a variety of acute and long-term health effects.

In response to these requests, NIOSH investigators conducted three onsite evaluations at Bally's, Paris, and Caesars Palace casinos. The first onsite evaluation was conducted July 22–24, 2005, during which we interviewed employees, reviewed OSHA Forms 200 and 300 (Log of Work Related Injuries and Illnesses), and administered a screening questionnaire. The screening questionnaire was used to select potential participants to take a subsequent health symptom questionnaire and undergo environmental and biological monitoring. During the second site visit, from August 21–24, 2005, additional screening questionnaires were distributed to NP casino dealers. A health symptom questionnaire was mailed January 6, 2006, and we conducted biological and environmental monitoring on our final site visit from January 19–22, 2006.

During the confidential medical interviews and the open discussions, NP casino dealers reported that they were most concerned about respiratory health effects related to ETS. NP casino dealers who worked in areas where smoking was permitted made up our study sample. Casino employees in administrative and engineering jobs who worked in areas where smoking was not permitted made up the comparison group. Of the responses from the health symptom questionnaire, the three most common symptoms reported by NP casino dealers were red or irritated eyes, cough, and stuffy nose. The prevalence of upper and lower respiratory symptoms, eye symptoms, headache, nausea, and dizziness was higher among the NP casino dealers than among the administrative and engineering employees, but these differences were not statistically significant. The low participation rate of the NP casino dealers and the small number of administrative and engineering casino employees may limit our ability to provide a confident estimate of symptom prevalence among these groups.

Of the 1,188 total poker and NP casino dealers working in Bally's, Paris, and Caesars Palace, 124 NP casino dealers participated in the environmental and/or biological exposure assessment. Full-shift PBZ and area air sampling for NIC, RSP, VOCs, PAHs, and ALD, were conducted in the casino gaming areas on Thursday, Friday, and Saturday during the swing shift and on Sunday during the day shift at all three casinos. We also monitored CO in the area samples.

NIC PBZ concentrations were similar to ranges found in a previous study of ETS in a casino. Of the 16 PAHs monitored, only naphthalene was present in quantifiable amounts. The VOCs identified included benzene, TOL, total hydrocarbons, p-dichlorobenzene, and limonene. The overall geometric means of the area samples were similar to those of the PBZ samples. Area CO concentrations were very low, with maximum values for each day measured ranging from 0.8–5.3 ppm in the three casinos.

We collected preshift and postshift urine samples on 114 NP casino dealers to determine whether levels of ETS biomarkers (COT and NNAL) in their urine would increase over an 8-hour work shift. Levels of NNAL in urine increased significantly during an 8-hour work shift both adjusting for, and not adjusting for, creatinine clearance. Creatinine-unadjusted COT increased during the 8-hour shift, but creatinine-adjusted COT decreased.

The NP casino dealers at Bally's, Paris, and Caesars Palace casinos had measurable airborne levels of ETS in their personal breathing zone and were found to absorb an ETS component into their bodies, as evidenced by measureable levels in the urine. The presence of NNAL in the urine demonstrates that casino dealers are exposed to a known carcinogen from the tobacco smoke. NP casino dealers reported higher prevalence of respiratory symptoms compared to administrative and engineering employees, but the differences in the prevalence between the groups were not statistically significant.

Keywords: NAICS 721120 (Casino Hotels), environmental tobacco smoke, ETS, nicotine, markers, respirable suspended particulates, formaldehyde, acetaldehyde, benzene, volatile organic compounds, naphthalene, cotinine, 4-(Methylnitrosoamino)-1-(3-pyridyl)-1-butanol, NNAL

INTRODUCTION

Between January and April 2005, NIOSH received confidential requests for HHEs from casino dealers at Bally's, Paris, and Caesars Palace casinos in Las Vegas, Nevada. NP casino dealers were concerned that exposure to ETS at work was causing a variety of health problems such as asthma, headaches, and eye irritation. NP casino dealers were also concerned about long-term health effects from ETS exposure such as cancer and heart disease. They also requested that the casino management provide gaming tables with built-in ventilation systems.

In response to these requests, NIOSH investigators conducted three onsite evaluations at Bally's, Paris, and Caesars Palace casinos. The first onsite evaluation was conducted July 22–24, 2005, during which we interviewed employees, reviewed OSHA Forms 200 and 300 (Log of Work Related Injuries and Illnesses) ("OSHA Logs") and administered a screening questionnaire to select potential participants for the health symptom questionnaire and environmental and biological monitoring. During the second site visit, from August 21–24, 2005, additional screening questionnaires were distributed to NP casino dealers. A health symptom questionnaire was mailed on January 6, 2006, to NP casino dealers and administrative staff, and we conducted biological and environmental monitoring on our final site visit January 19–22, 2006. At the start of the evaluation, Caesars Entertainment owned the casinos; by the January 2006 visit, Harrah's Entertainment owned them.

Of the three casinos, Caesars Palace is the largest (129,000 square feet), followed by Paris (83,000 square feet), and Bally's (67,000 square feet). Each of the casinos offers table gaming such as blackjack, poker, roulette, and craps. Gaming tables are usually arranged to form an oval, called a "pit." At the time of our first site visit, smoking was permitted for patrons throughout the gaming area of the three casinos except for poker tables in Bally's casino. By our third visit, Caesars Palace had established a smoke-free poker room. Employees on the gaming floors include casino dealers, pit supervisors, cocktail servers, security officers, and managers. Most of the Bally's, Paris, and Caesars Palace casino dealers worked throughout the gaming areas where smoking was permitted, but at the time of our site visits, a small percentage of casino dealers worked only at the poker tables where smoking was not permitted. Work schedules are similar at the three casinos. The casinos are open 24 hours a day, and casino dealers primarily work one of several 8-hour shifts.

Our comparison group included casino employees assigned to administrative and engineering job duties who worked in areas of the casinos where smoking was not permitted, adjacent to the casino gaming areas and with separate ventilation. Administrative and engineering employees worked 8-hour daytime shifts, 5 days a week. We included the comparison group to provide a background prevalence of symptoms to which the prevalence of symptoms among the exposed group (NP casino dealers) could be compared.

Assessment

The principal objectives of these HHEs were to quantify NP casino dealers' exposure to ETS and to determine the prevalence of respiratory symptoms among NP casino dealers. To achieve these objectives, the evaluation was conducted in three phases. During the preliminary assessment phase, July 22–24 and August 21–24, 2005, we interviewed employees, reviewed OSHA Logs, and administered a screening questionnaire to select potential participants for the subsequent phases of the study. In the second phase, January 6, 2006, we mailed a health symptom questionnaire to NP casino dealers and casino employees in administrative and engineering jobs. In the third phase, January 19–22, 2006, we assessed levels of NIC, 4-VP, RSP/SOL, TOL, THC, PAHs, VOCs, and ALDs (FLD and ACLTD) in the air, and levels of COT, NNAL, and creatinine in the urine of NP casino dealers over an 8-hour shift.

Preliminary Assessment

Employee Interviews and Review of OSHA Logs

During the initial site visit (July 2005), casino dealers at Bally's, Paris, and Caesars Palace casinos were invited to discuss their health concerns in a private room with one of three NIOSH medical officers. These interviews were scheduled so that employees working any shift had an opportunity to speak with the medical officers. Many of the dealers also openly discussed their health concerns in the dealer break rooms where medical officers were available.

The OSHA Logs were reviewed for the years 2003–2005 for Bally's and Paris casinos. For Caesars Palace, the OSHA Logs from 1999, 2000, 2001, 2003, and 2004 were reviewed; OSHA Logs for 2002 were not available. Information from the employee interviews and the OSHA Logs was used in designing the health symptom questionnaire. A summary of the employee interviews and review of OSHA Logs appears in Appendix A.

Selection of Potential Study Participants

Based on employee records provided by casino management, 1,188 poker and NP casino dealers were working at the time of our evaluation. This number included 211 dealers at Bally's, 319 dealers at Paris, 545 dealers at Caesars Palace, and 113 dealers who worked on an as-needed basis (extra board dealers) for Bally's and Paris casinos. No information was available on the number of workers unexposed to ETS at the three casinos.

During the July and August 2005 site visits, NIOSH investigators used a screening questionnaire to identify potential study participants for the health symptom questionnaire and biological and environmental monitoring. Participation in the screening questionnaire was open to all casino employees who worked in the gaming areas of the casinos, as well as administrative and engineering employees who worked in locations adjacent to the casino gaming areas that had separate ventilation. We distributed screening questionnaires in gaming employees' break rooms where casino dealers and other casino gaming employees began their work shift and took breaks. Although other casino employees from the gaming floor used the break rooms, we narrowed our selection and targeted only NP casino dealers for participation in the subsequent phases of the study. We distributed the screening questionnaire to administrative and engineering employees at their workstations. After completing the questionnaires, employees returned them to locked boxes, directly to NIOSH investigators, or by mail in NIOSH-provided, addressed, stamped envelopes. Of the 467 casino employees who returned screening questionnaires, 412 were from employees working in smoking permitted areas, and 55 were from employees in the areas of the casinos that do not permit smoking.

The screening questionnaire asked employees for contact information, sex, date of birth, job title, name of casino they worked in, and work shift. It also asked whether they currently smoke or use tobacco products and whether they live with someone who smokes inside the home. Employees were selected as potential study participants for the health symptom questionnaire and the biological and environmental monitoring if they reported they did not use any tobacco products and were not living with someone who smokes inside the home. We found 365 employees who met these initial inclusion criteria for the health symptom questionnaire and biological and environmental monitoring.

Air Sampling (July 2005)

Full-shift area air sampling for NIC, RSP, VOCs, CO, and PAHs was conducted in the casino gaming areas during the swing shifts at all three casinos. These samples were used to work out logistical issues pertaining to sample collection and to develop analytical methods for SOL (extracted from the RSP sample filters) and 4-VP (extracted from the XAD-4™ sorbent tubes used to collect NIC). Because the samples were not collected to provide information on human exposure to ETS and were not part of the HHE requests, this report does not discuss these results.

Ventilation Overview

NIOSH investigators reviewed casino ventilation diagrams and discussed them with the casinos' facility engineers. These findings are available in Appendix B. No ventilation measurements were taken by NIOSH investigators at any of the casinos.

Health Symptom Questionnaire

Health symptom questionnaires and stamped return envelopes were mailed to 365 casino employees who met our initial inclusion criteria from the screening questionnaire. The questionnaire was mailed January 6, 2006, prior to our on-site exposure assessment January 19–22, 2006.

Employees were asked if they have ever smoked or currently smoke tobacco products, lived with someone who smokes inside the home, or were exposed more than 5 days per week to tobacco smoke in other settings, such as in bars, restaurants, or other places. Employees were also asked for job type, number of hours they worked in a week, and name of the casino where they worked. Only NP casino dealers and administrative and engineering casino employees were included in the analysis of the questionnaire data. Additionally, employees were included in the analyses for the health symptom questionnaire if they reported no current use of tobacco products, did not live with someone who smokes inside the home, and had no exposure to tobacco smoke more than 5 days per week in other settings such as bars, restaurants, or other places.

ASSESSMENT
(CONTINUED)

Participants were asked if they had experienced respiratory symptoms, eye symptoms, dizziness, headache, or nausea in the last 4 weeks while working in the casino(s). A participant's symptom was defined as work-related if it improved on days away from work. Participants were determined to have current asthma if a physician had diagnosed them with asthma and they indicated in the questionnaire that they still had asthma. Symptoms consistent with work-related asthma were defined as the presence of work-related wheeze, or two or more of the following symptoms: work-related cough, chest tightness, or shortness of breath.

Exposure Assessment

Additional inclusion criteria for participants in the biological monitoring and environmental assessment phases were as follows: (1) participants had to be NP casino dealers and (2) they had to work either the swing shift (starts between 6 p.m. and 9 p.m.) from Thursday through Saturday, or the day shift (starts between 9 a.m. and 12 p m.) on Sunday. These shift/time combinations were identified by NP casino dealers as the busiest times of the week, possibly when ETS levels were highest. We identified 213 NP casino dealers as potential participants for the biological and environmental monitoring using these additional criteria.

Biological Monitoring

On the days of the exposure assessment, we verbally administered an acute exposure questionnaire. We asked the NP casino dealers about their use of tobacco products, how long ago they used tobacco products, whether they use NRT, exposure to ETS in the 4 days prior to sampling, the casino they worked in, and the shift they worked. As an additional step, we verbally verified that participants were nonsmokers. To participate in the biological monitoring, NP casino dealers had to report no current use of tobacco products and no ETS exposure outside of work. For NP casino dealers who reported NRT use, analysis of biological monitoring was restricted to NNAL.

From among the 213 NP casino dealers who were potential participants, we chose a convenience sample of 124 participants for biological monitoring. This number of participants was chosen to match the limited number of PBZ air sampling pumps available for these participants to wear during the evaluation. We targeted 10 NP casino dealers at each casino on each day that we conducted biological monitoring. NP casino dealers provided a urine sample before the start of their work shift and at the end of the work shift. NIOSH investigators provided them with urine cups to collect their samples. The samples were analyzed for urinary COT, total NNAL, and creatinine (used to adjust for urinary dilution). Individual results for the biological monitoring component were mailed to participants.

COT is the major metabolite of NIC with a biological half-life of approximately 16–20 hours. The biological half-life is the time required for a substance within a biological system to decrease by one half. The rate of removal is often approximately exponential. When detected in the urine, COT provides a valuable indicator of tobacco smoke exposure, including secondary smoke exposure from the previous 1–2 days [Pirkle et al. 1996]. The tobacco-specific nitrosamine NNAL is a urinary metabolite of NNK, which is a potent pulmonary carcinogen in humans. NNK is not found in materials other than tobacco, so the presence of NNAL provides a direct association between tobacco exposure and body burden of a tobacco-related carcinogen [Benowitz 1999]. In one study that quantified urinary levels of NNK and NNAL in cigarette smokers after smoking cessation, the researchers estimated that NNAL had an elimination half- life of 45.2 days and that NNK had an elimination half-life of 39.6 days [Hecht et al. 1999]. No research is available describing the elimination of NNK and its metabolites as a result of exposure to ETS. The methods used for these analyses are available in Appendix C.

Environmental Monitoring

Full-shift area and PBZ air samples for NIC, 4-VP, RSP/SOL, TOL, THC, PAHs, VOCs, and ALDs (FLD and ACTLD) were collected at each casino. The specific sampling and analytical methods for these analytes are available in Appendix C. We collected two sets of area samples daily at each casino. The purpose of the area samples was to continuously monitor the ambient concentrations in the gaming areas for worst-case exposure scenarios, and to see how they compared with PBZ sample measures. Area samplers were placed within the center of the pit and at the same height as the PBZ of the dealers. Ambient parameters, such as temperature, RH, and CO_2 concentration, as well as CO concentration (found in ETS from tobacco combustion), were measured using a QTRAK Plus®, a direct reading instrument (TSI, St. Paul, Minnesota). Background information on ETS, such as health effects, as well as OELs on environmental measures that were collected, are available in Appendix D.

PBZ air samples were collected on 10 NP casino dealers at each casino who provided urine samples each day. If these dealers opted not to wear the sampling equipment, we attempted to recruit new nonsmoking NP casino dealers to replace them. Because the NIOSH staging areas were where NP casino dealers reported to work, we were able to efficiently recruit new participants, verify that they met the inclusion criteria to participate, and enroll them into the environmental and biological monitoring. We then collected their preshift urine sample and provided them with environmental samplers prior to the start of their work shift. All NP casino dealers who contributed a urine sample were asked to wear samplers for NIC and 4-VP; eight of the ten NP casino dealers were also asked to wear an additional sampler that would sample for one of the following: RSP/SOL, PAH, and VOCs. The remaining two NP casino dealers were asked to wear a badge that passively measured ALD in the air. In a few instances, volunteers wearing the samplers for RSP/SOL, PAH, and VOCs requested passive badges to measure their ALD exposures. Whenever possible we provided them with these badges. Specific analytical methods for each of these analytes are available in Appendix C.

Statistical Analysis

We used SAS version 9.1 (SAS Institute, Cary, North Carolina) for all statistical analyses. Using chi-square tests and Fisher's exact tests at a significance level of 0.05, we compared the prevalence of symptoms between NP casino dealers and casino workers in administrative and engineering jobs. Symptoms considered included respiratory symptoms, eye irritation, sore throat, headache, nausea, and dizziness. We also examined the differences between preshift and postshift NNAL, NNAL adjusted for creatinine, COT, and COT adjusted for creatinine using paired t-tests or paired signed tests, depending on the distributions of the differences. Pearson's or Spearman's correlation coefficients were calculated among and between environmental and biological sampling results.

For environmental and NNAL samples with mass below the LOD, an estimate of the mass was obtained by dividing the LOD (obtained from the laboratory) by $\sqrt{2}$. Hornung and Reed [1990] have described this method of handling censored data. For the environmental samples, this estimate was divided by the maximum sample volume to obtain the estimated sample concentration. The MDCs were determined by dividing the LOD by the maximum sample volume. Similarly, where the lab did not report COT measures below the LOQ, the LOQ divided by $\sqrt{2}$ was used.

RESULTS

Health Symptom Questionnaire

NIOSH investigators mailed 365 health symptom questionnaires to participants who met inclusion criteria based on responses to the screening questionnaire; of these, 195 (53%) completed and returned the questionnaire. After reviewing the responses, we determined that 36 participants did not meet our inclusion criteria for the health symptom questionnaire; they were removed from the analysis. This resulted in 159 participants who met the inclusion criteria for the health symptom questionnaire, 147 NP casino dealers and 12 administrative or engineering casino employees. The mean age of the NP casino dealers was 48 years (range: 24–73); 79 (54%) were women. The mean age of the administrative and engineering casino employees was 48 years (range: 27–67); 8 (67%) were women. Table 1 shows the number of participants in the health symptom questionnaire by casino and job group. The mean number of hours worked across all three casinos was 41 hours (range: 5–80) for NP casino dealers and 43 hours (range: 40–55) for administrative and engineering casino employees.

Table 1. Number of participants by casino for health symptom questionnaire

Casino	NP casino dealers	Administrative and engineering casino employees
	n	n
Bally's only	23	2
Paris only	48	5
Caesars Palace only	62	0
Multiple casinos*	14	5
Total	147	12

*Fourteen dealers and five administrative and engineering employees reported working at two or more casinos.

RESULTS
(CONTINUED)

Table 2 presents the prevalences of work-related symptoms for the NP casino dealers and the administrative and engineering casino employees. The three most common health symptoms reported by the NP casino dealers were red or irritated eyes (49%), cough (48%), and stuffy nose (43%). The prevalences of respiratory symptoms, eye symptoms, headache, nausea, and dizziness were higher among the NP casino dealers than among the administrative and engineering casino employees, but these differences were not statistically significant.

Table 2. Prevalences of work-related health symptoms* in participants

Health Symptom	NP casino dealers n(%)[†]	Administrative and engineering casino employees n (%)[‡]	p value
Red or irritated eyes	68 (49)	4 (33)	0.31
Cough	68 (48)	3 (25)	0.13
Stuffy nose	60 (43)	3 (25)	0.36
Sneezing	59 (42)	2 (17)	0.13
Runny nose	57 (40)	2 (17)	0.13
Itching eyes	54 (39)	2 (17)	0.21
Headache	51 (37)	2 (17)	0.22
Watery eyes	47 (33)	2 (17)	0.34
Sore or scratchy throat	43 (31)	1 (8)	0.18
Shortness of breath	25 (17)	1 (8)	0.69
Dizziness	23 (16)	0	0.22
Wheezing or whistling in chest	21 (14)	0	0.37
Tightness in chest	18 (13)	0	0.36
Nausea	11 (8)	0	1.00

*Report of symptom in the last 4 weeks while working in a casino and positive response to "Does this symptom improve on your days off?"
[†]Denominators vary from 139–145.
[‡]Denominator is 12.

Table 3 presents the prevalence of current physician-diagnosed asthma and symptoms that suggest work-related asthma in NP casino dealers and administrative and engineering casino employees. The prevalences of symptoms that suggest work-related asthma were higher among the NP casino dealers than among the administrative and engineering casino employees, but the differences were not statistically significant. Of the 11 NP casino dealers who reported they had current physician-diagnosed asthma, seven reported their asthma was worse when they were at work.

Table 3. Prevalence of physician-diagnosed asthma and symptoms that suggest asthma in participants

	NP casino dealers n (%)*	Administrative and engineering casino employees n (%)[†]	p value
Current physician-diagnosed asthma[‡]	11 (8)	2 (20)	0.22
Symptoms suggestive of work-related asthma[§]	35 (24)	0	0.07

*Denominators range from 122–143.
[†]Denominators range from 8–12.
[‡]Asthma was reported as being diagnosed by a physician and a positive response to "Do you still have asthma?"
[§]Reported the presence of work-related wheeze, or two of the following three symptoms: work-related cough, work-related chest tightness, or work-related shortness of breath.

Exposure Assessment

Environmental Monitoring

Tables 4 and 5 present the geometric means, sample sizes, and ranges for the PBZ and area air samples by casino and for all casinos combined. The GMs of the area and PBZ sample concentrations were comparable within casinos for a particular analyte.

Table 4. Geometric means (sample sizes) and ranges of ETS components (µg/m³) in PBZ air samples

	Bally's GM (n)	Range	Paris GM (n)	Range	Caesars Palace GM (n)	Range	Combined GM (n)	Range
ACTLD	9.30 (11)	6.2–15	9.16 (12)	4.8–16	15.1 (6)	14–17	10.2 (29)	4.8–17
4-VP	0.867 (34)	0.18–2.8	0.852 (35)	0.18–1.7	1.33 (38)	0.57–2.5	1.00 (107)	0.18–2.8
FLD	7.46 (11)	2.3–22	7.75 (12)	2.3–29	16.8 (6)	14–23	8.96 (29)	2.3–29
NIC	4.60 (34)	1.6–12	4.03 (35)	0.58–10	7.80 (38)	3.9–17	5.32 (107)	0.58–17
PAH*	0.652 (12)	0.21–1.2	0.753 (11)	0.25–1.2	1.02 (11)	0.72–1.4	0.790 (34)	0.21–1.4
RSP	43.0 (11)	22–78	31.6 (10)	13–56	52.5 (12)	13–140	42.1 (33)	13–140
SOL	0.208 (11)	0.07–0.82	0.145 (10)	0.07–0.55	0.352 (12)	0.07–1.1	0.226 (33)	0.07–1.1
THC	208 (6)	56–390	425 (7)	130–1200	735 (9)	230–3100	438 (22)	56–3100
TOL	23.1 (6)	5.6–290	6.29 (7)	5.6–13	18.5 (9)	5.6–180	13.9 (22)	5.6–290

*The concentrations reflect the levels of naphthalene, the only PAH detected in the samples.

Table 5. Geometric means (sample sizes), and ranges of ETS components (µg/m³) in area air samples

	Bally's GM (n)	Range	Paris GM (n)	Range	Caesars Palace GM (n)	Range	Combined GM (n)	Range
ACTLD	8.55 (5)	2.3–19	9.30 (8)	6.9–14	15.4 (6)	7.6–20	11.0 (19)	2.3–20
4-VP	0.831 (8)	0.18–1.8	1.10 (8)	0.72–1.6	1.76 (8)	0.97–3.4	1.20 (24)	0.18–3.4
FLD	7.19 (5)	2.3–36	6.70 (8)	2.3–14	15.6 (6)	7.6–34	8.91 (19)	2.3–36
NIC	5.31 (8)	1.0–14	5.31 (8)	2.6–7.2	10.7 (8)	4.5–23	6.69 (24)	1.0–23
PAH*	0.607 (7)	0.31–1.2	0.617 (8)	0.19–1.3	1.01 (8)	0.55–1.6	0.729 (23)	0.19–1.6
RSP	38.1 (6)	23–77	32.6 (8)	25–44	56.1 (8)	40–86	41.4 (22)	23–86
SOL	0.300 (6)	0.07–0.89	0.141 (8)	0.07–0.36	0.359 (8)	0.10–0.99	0.242 (22)	0.07–0.99
THC	320 (8)	142–470	251 (8)	130–420	553 (8)	200–960	354 (24)	130–960
TOL	18.7 (8)	5.6–500	6.61 (8)	5.6–12	9.56 (8)	5.6–19	10.6 (24)	5.6–500

*The concentrations reflect the levels of naphthalene, the only PAH detected in the samples.

Nicotine and 4-Vinyl Pyridine

The MDCs for NIC and 4-VP, based on a sample volume of 765 liters, were 0.26 µg/m³. None of the PBZ NIC measures and three of the PBZ 4-VP measures were below the MDC. PBZ concentrations ranged from 0.58 to 17 µg/m³ for NIC and from below the MDC to 2.8 µg/m³ for 4-VP. For all three casinos combined, the geometric mean for PBZ NIC was 5.32 µg/m³ and 1.00 µg/m³ for 4-VP.

None of the NIC area measures and only one 4-VP measure was below the MDC. Area measures for NIC ranged from 1.0 to 23 µg/m³; the 4-VP concentrations ranged from below the MDC to 3.4 µg/m³. For all three casinos combined, the geometric mean for area NIC was 6.69 µg/m³ and 1.20 µg/m³ for 4-VP.

Polynuclear Aromatic Hydrocarbons

Of the 16 PAHs analyzed, only naphthalene was detected in quantifiable concentrations. All naphthalene PBZ measures were above the MDC. PBZ concentrations of naphthalene ranged from 0.21 to 1.4 µg/m³. The geometric mean for all three casinos combined for PBZ naphthalene was 0.790 µg/m³. Of the 24 area measures taken, one was not analyzed because of pump failure. The remaining 23 area measures ranged from 0.19 to 1.6 µg/m³. The geometric mean for area naphthalene samples for all three casinos combined was 0.729 µg/m³.

Respirable Suspended Particulates and Solanesol

Based on a sample volume of 1056 liters, the MDC for RSP was 19 µg/m³ and 0.09 µg/m³ for SOL. Three PBZ measures for RSP and eleven PBZ measures for SOL were below the MDC. PBZ concentrations ranged from below the MDC to 140 µg/m³ for RSP and from below the MDC to 1.1 µg/m³ for SOL. For all three casinos combined, the geometric mean for RSP was 42.1 µg/m³ and 0.226 µg/m³ for SOL.

None of the area RSP measures and six SOL measures was below the MDC. Two RSP/SOL area samples were damaged during shipping and were not analyzed. Area measures for RSP ranged from 23 to 86 µg/m³; area SOL measures ranged from below the MDC to 0.99 µg/m³. For all three casinos combined, the geometric mean for area RSP was 41.4 µg/m³ and 0.242 µg/m³ for SOL.

Volatile Organic Compounds

A VOC screen using thermal desorption tubes indicated the presence of approximately 98 chemicals per sample in the air;

approximately 20 of these chemicals are commonly found in indoor environments. The chemicals were analyzed using gas chromatography with mass spectrometry detection. Figure 1 shows a typical profile of the VOCs present in the casinos. The x-axis denotes the retention time of a compound, i.e., the time taken to separate from a mixture of chemicals. The y-axis is a measure of total ion abundances at the retention times. Each scan per second made by the analytical instrument is plotted as a point (time, abundance) forming the ion chromatogram. Abundance is a measure of concentration, i.e., the higher the ion abundance, the higher the amount of analyte present. The actual abundance "numbers" are relative to what scale is chosen for the plot.

Figure 1. Profile of chemicals inside casinos

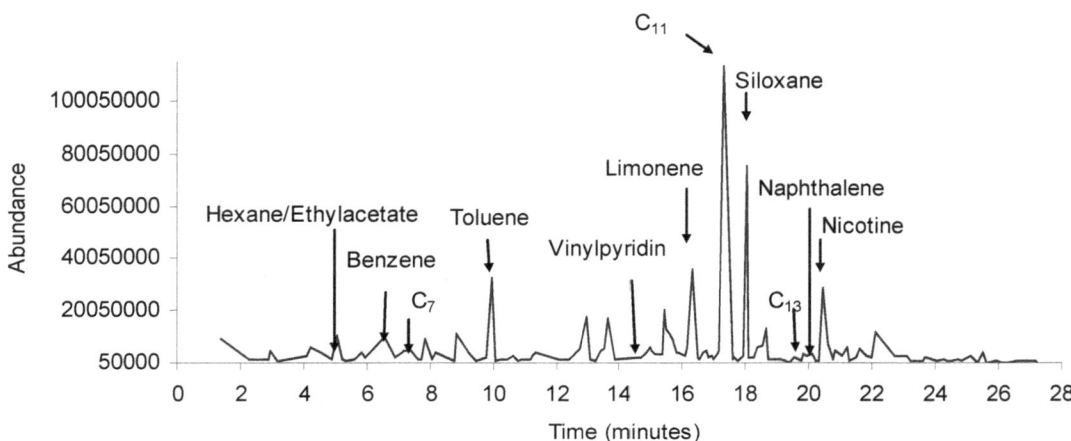

Only compounds with an abundance above the threshold limit of the analytical instrument were included in this figure. Based on this profile, benzene, TOL, p-dichlorobenzene, limonene, and THC were chosen for quantitative analysis based on the relative amount present in the environment, their relative toxicities compared to other VOCs, and ability to separate them from the mixture. A trace concentration of p-dichlorobenzene was found in one PBZ sample at Bally's. Quantifiable concentrations of benzene were found in two PBZ samples, both at Caesars Palace. The full-shift concentrations for both samples were 12 ppb and 13 ppb. Quantifiable concentrations of limonene were found in two PBZ samples at Bally's (0.6 mg/m^3 and 1.3 mg/m^3) and in four PBZ samples at Caesars Palace (0.1 mg/m^3, 0.1 mg/m^3, 0.9 mg/m^3, and 1.0 mg/m^3).

Based on a sample volume of 51 liters, the MDC for TOL was 8 µg/m^3 and 79 µg/m^3 for THC. Thirteen TOL PBZ measures and one THC PBZ measure were below the MDC. The PBZ concentrations of TOL ranged from below the MDC to 290 µg/m³, and the PBZ concentrations of THC ranged from below the MDC to 3100 µg/m³. The geometric mean in the PBZ measures at all three casinos combined was 13.9 µg/m³ for TOL and 438 µg/m³ for THC. Fourteen of the 24 area measures for TOL and none of the THC measures were below the MDC. Area TOL measures ranged from below the MDC to 500 µg/m³, and area THC measures ranged from 130 to 960 µg/m³. The geometric mean in the area measures for all three casinos combined was 10.6 µg/m³ for TOL and 354 µg/m³ for THC.

Formaldehyde and Acetaldehyde

The MDCs for FLD and ACTLD based on a sample volume of 16 liters were 3.2 µg/m³. Five of the FLD measures and none of the ACTLD PBZ measures were below the MDC. PBZ concentrations ranged from below the MDC to 29 µg/m³ for formaldehyde, and from 4.8 to 17 µg/m³ for ACTLD. For all three casinos combined, the geometric mean for PBZ FLD was 8.96 µg/m³ and 10.2 µg/m³ for ACTLD. Five ALD area samples were damaged during shipping and were not analyzed. Of the 19 samples that were analyzed, three FLD and one ACTLD area measures were below the MDC. The area concentrations of FLD ranged from below the MDC to 36 µg/m³, and the area concentrations for ACTLD ranged from below the MDC to 20 µg/m³. The highest area concentrations of FLD (36 µg/m³) and ACTLD (20 µg/m³) were collected on the same sample. For all three casinos, the geometric mean for area FLD was 8.91 µg/m³ and 11.0 µg/m³ for ACTLD.

Carbon Monoxide

CO measures collected at 1-minute intervals were mostly below the instrument's detection limit of 0.1 ppm. The maximum readings at the three casinos for each of the 4 days measured ranged from 0.8–5.3 ppm.

Temperature, Relative Humidity, and Carbon Dioxide

Temperature and RH values were within the ASHRAE ranges for acceptable human comfort, except on one instance in the Paris casino, where the temperature was below the ASHRAE indoor design guidance of 68.5°F for winter temperatures [ANSI/ASHRAE 2004]. At each casino, maximum CO_2 concentrations were more than 700 ppm above the outdoor CO_2 concentrations suggesting that not enough outdoor air may have been provided for acceptable odor control (body odor) and indicating the need for further evaluation of the ventilation systems, as discussed in Appendix D. The outdoor CO_2 concentrations ranged from 250–300 ppm. Table 6 summarizes these results.

Table 6. Ranges of indoor environmental quality parameters

Casino	Temperature (°F)	RH (%)	CO_2 (ppm)
Bally's	69.4–74.3	12.4–18.7	450–1311
Paris	60.5–74.7	8.3–18.9	286–1220
Caesars Palace	69.3–77.0	9.6–23.1	583–1244

Biological Monitoring

Of 213 NP casino dealers, 124 (58%) participated in the biological monitoring portion of the evaluation. All verbally reported they were nonsmokers, and 107 (86%) participants reported they had been exposed to ETS at work in the last 4 days. Of the 483 urine samples (123 COT and 122 NNAL preshift and 119 COT and 119 NNAL postshift), some measures from four participants were excluded from the analysis. Two participants were removed because they reported on the exposure questionnaire that they were exposed to tobacco smoke in a bar or other setting in the past 4 days. One participant was removed because of a COT value inconsistent with being a nonsmoker. One participant was not included in the COT analysis because of reported use of NRT. Other sampling issues included a lack of both a preshift and postshift sample and insufficient sample volume for COT, NNAL, and creatinine. For the purposes of the comparative analysis, this resulted in 114 preshift and postshift (paired) samples for unadjusted COT and NNAL, and 112 preshift and postshift (paired) samples for creatinine-adjusted COT. A sample size of 113 preshift and postshift (paired) samples of creatinine-adjusted NNAL was used for the comparative analysis. Fourteen COT measures were below the LOQ of 10 ng/mL and 93 NNAL measures were below the LOD of 0.0030 ng/mL. Of the 93 NNAL measures, 63 (68%) below the LOD were in the preshift samples, and 30 of the 93 (32%) NNAL measures below the LOD were in the postshift samples.

Table 7 presents the geometric mean levels of preshift and postshift COT and NNAL for each casino and for all casinos combined unadjusted for creatinine. Table 8 presents the geometric mean levels of preshift and postshift COT and NNAL adjusted for creatinine.

RESULTS
(CONTINUED)

Table 7. Geometric means (and sample size) of creatinine-unadjusted ETS components in urine

| Casino | COT (ng/mL) | | NNAL (ng/mL) | |
	Preshift GM (n)	Postshift GM (n)	Preshift GM (n)	Postshift GM (n)
Bally's	27.55 (34)	34.18 (34)	0.0053 (35)	0.0089 (35)
Paris	19.30 (35)	25.92 (35)	0.0042 (35)	0.0079 (35)
Caesars Palace	21.15 (45)	31.41 (45)	0.0029 (44)	0.0050 (44)
Combined	22.25 (114)	30.37 (114)	0.0039 (114)	0.0069 (114)

Table 8. Geometric means (and sample size) of creatinine-adjusted ETS components in urine

| Casino | COT (nmol/mgcr) | | NNAL (pmol/mgcr) | |
	Preshift GM (n)	Postshift GM (n)	Preshift GM (n)	Postshift GM (n)
Bally's	0.1706 (34)	0.1640 (34)	0.0270 (35)	0.0353 (35)
Paris	0.1302 (34)	0.1192 (34)	0.0236 (35)	0.0297 (35)
Caesars Palace	0.1947 (44)	0.1778 (44)	0.0226 (43)	0.0242 (43)
Combined	0.1655 (112)	0.1536 (112)	0.0242 (113)	0.0290 (113)

Because the pattern of biological monitoring results was similar across casinos, our analysis focused on the combined results. Urinary COT and NNAL levels unadjusted for creatinine for all three casinos combined increased significantly during an 8-hour shift ($p < 0.01$). The levels of urinary NNAL adjusted for creatinine for all three casinos combined increased significantly over an 8-hour shift ($p = 0.03$). However, urinary COT levels adjusted for creatinine for all three casinos combined decreased over an 8-hour shift. The preshift urinary COT was positively correlated with preshift urinary NNAL ($r = 0.55$, $p < 0.01$) and postshift urinary COT was positively correlated with postshift urinary NNAL levels ($r = 0.55$, $p < 0.01$). The net urinary NNAL correlated with the net COT ($r = 0.49$; $p < 0.01$). The net levels of NNAL and COT correspond to their preshift level subtracted from their postshift level. All correlations were calculated using NNAL and COT levels that were unadjusted for creatinine.

Relationship between Biological and Environmental Measures of ETS Exposure

No statistically significant positive correlations were found between the concentrations of unadjusted and adjusted NNAL and environmental measures (NIC, 4-VP, RSP/SOL, PAHs, TOL, THC, FLD, ACTLD) during the 4-day evaluation. No statistically significant positive correlation was found between unadjusted COT and environmental measures (NIC, 4-VP, RSP/SOL,

PAHs, TOL, THC, FLD, ACTLD) over the 4-day evaluation. No statistically significant positive correlation was found between adjusted COT and most of the environmental measures (NIC, 4-VP, TOL, THC, FLD, ACTLD) except for the following environmental measures: PAH (0.40), RSP (0.58), and SOL (0.42) where we found a statistically significant positive correlation.

DISCUSSION

In this evaluation we found that NP casino dealers were exposed to workplace ETS, and that they absorbed detectable ETS-specific components, including a tobacco-specific carcinogen, into their bodies. The 2006 U.S. Surgeon General's Report concluded that the presence of NNAL in urine links ETS exposure with an increased risk of lung cancer in nonsmokers, and that exposure to ETS causes lung cancer. The report further concludes that no risk-free level of exposure to ETS exists and that eliminating smoking in indoor spaces fully protects nonsmokers from exposure to ETS. Other methods to reduce exposure, such as separating smokers from nonsmokers, cleaning the air, and ventilating buildings, cannot eliminate exposures of nonsmokers to ETS [DHHS 2006]. Although past research has demonstrated that ETS is harmful to those who are occupationally exposed, we chose to conduct a comprehensive evaluation because of the lack of biological monitoring and health effect data specifically on casino dealers who are exposed to ETS in the workplace.

Environmental Monitoring

The findings from this evaluation are consistent with those found in other ETS exposure assessment studies. The range of PBZ NIC air sample concentrations (0.58–17 μg/m³) is comparable to past studies of workers in smoking environments [Phillips et al. 1998; Jenkins and Counts 1999], including one study of casino dealers [Trout et al. 1998]. Likewise, the range of area air sample concentrations of NIC was comparable to data reported by Trout et al. [1998], who reported PBZ NIC concentrations between 6 and 15 μg/m³ for casino dealers. The area air concentrations in this study were similar to the PBZ sample concentrations, indicating that they were representative of the overall atmosphere in the casino pits.

DISCUSSION
(CONTINUED)

Historically, RSP has been used as a surrogate for the particulate phase of ETS. RSP is easy to quantify in the environment. A drawback is that it is not specific to ETS, thus possibly leading to an overestimation of ETS levels. The maximum area RSP level in this evaluation was 86 $\mu g/m^3$, which is similar to the 90 $\mu g/m^3$ reported by Trout et al. [1998]. The highest PBZ RSP concentration in this evaluation was 140 $\mu g/m^3$; Trout et al. [1998] did not measure PBZ RSP levels. In addition to RSP, SOL, a trisesquiterpenoid alcohol found in tobacco leaves, has been used as a surrogate for ETS components in the particulate phase [Ogden and Maiolo 1989; Tang et al. 1990]. However, recent research suggests that SOL is degraded in indoor environments with ozone concentrations of 40 ppb [Tucker and Pretty 2005]. Ozone levels were not measured as part of this evaluation.

A surprising finding from this evaluation was that common PAHs, such as benzo-a-pyrene, anthracene, or pyrene, were not found in the PBZ and area air samples. These compounds, some of which are known lung carcinogens, have been found in previous studies of ETS in homes and restaurants [Husgafvel-Pursiainen et al. 1986; Grimmer and Naujack 1987]. Of the 16 PAHs evaluated, only naphthalene was found in quantifiable concentrations in both PBZ and area air samples. The EPA has classified naphthalene as a possible human carcinogen [EPA 2008]. Overall, the concentrations of TOL, FLD, and ACTLD were lower than those reported in the scientific literature, although past ETS studies of these compounds were conducted in smaller spaces such as restaurants, automobiles, and residences.

Although the airborne components were below applicable regulatory and recommended OELs for these components individually, studies have shown that simultaneous exposure to multiple components (mixed exposures), even at low levels, can cause respiratory health effects, such as acute bronchitis and asthma [Burnett et al. 1994; Sheppard et al. 1999; Pope 2000]. These studies focused on health effects from air pollution from non-ETS fine particulates, but the mixed-exposure effects seen in these studies are still relevant to ETS exposure because many air pollutants (RSP, PAHs, VOCs, and ALDs) are also found in ETS. The regulatory and recommended OELs for these components are based on the individual component; the synergistic or additive properties are not considered [Lippy and Turner 1991]. OELs for some chemicals found in ETS (such as NIC) were developed to protect workers whose exposure (route and quantity) to these chemicals are different from the ETS exposure route, as discussed in Appendix D.

Most of the temperature and RH values measured during this evaluation fell within the acceptable ranges of thermal comfort recommended by ASHRAE. Each ventilation system reportedly was designed to comply with the relevant outdoor air recommendations in effect at the time of their installation. However, our limited area air monitoring data showed indoor concentrations of CO_2 to be more than 700 ppm relative to outdoors, suggesting the need to further evaluate the effectiveness of the ventilation systems in maintaining acceptable odor control. [It should be noted that this guideline refers to the control of body odor from sedentary people and not odor from tobacco smoke.] As discussed in Appendix B, two of the casinos (Paris and Caesars Palace) had CO_2 sensors in the ductwork, but we do not know if the relationships between duct concentrations and breathing zone concentrations have been evaluated or if these sensors have been calibrated or maintained properly. The concentrations of ETS compounds could be expected to be higher when less outdoor air is brought into the casinos, and lower with more outdoor air to dilute these contaminants. ASHRAE has a position document stating that, although implementing engineering controls, such as current and advanced dilution ventilation, can reduce odors and some forms of irritation from ETS, it should not be relied upon to control health risks from ETS exposure in public spaces. ASHRAE concludes that the only means of eliminating the health risks associated with indoor ETS exposure is to ban all smoking [ASHRAE 2005].

Biological Monitoring

The biological monitoring portion of the evaluation was designed to evaluate body burden of ETS metabolites; that is, whether the ETS components were absorbed in the body, metabolized, and detectable in the urine. Biological monitoring has been commonly used to assess ETS exposure by measuring COT in the serum or urine of exposed persons. Because COT is the major metabolite of NIC, it has been extensively used in large epidemiological studies to measure exposure to ETS. However, COT is potentially problematic in that levels can be affected by the ingestion of NIC-containing foods and beverages, and it is not a specific indicator relevant to potential carcinogenicity [Benowitz 1999; Hecht 2002]. The tobacco-specific nitrosamine, NNK, along with its urinary metabolite NNAL, are known pulmonary carcinogens [Hecht

2002], and the presence of NNAL in urine links ETS exposure with an increased risk of lung cancer, a long-term outcome of ETS exposure [DHHS 2006]. NNAL is a tobacco-specific compound, so its detection specifically indicates ETS exposure [Hecht 2002]. The differences in NNAL and COT may help to explain the low correlation between NNAL and COT seen in this evaluation.

We have documented an increase in urinary levels of NNAL over a work shift in casino dealers, which provides strong evidence that the increase is due to workplace ETS exposure. Our results are consistent with other studies that have shown an increase in levels of NNAL in bar and restaurant workers exposed to ETS over a work shift and casino patrons exposed over a 4-hour period [Parsons et al. 1998; Anderson et al. 2003; Stark et al. 2007].

We have reported COT and NNAL levels with and without creatinine adjustment. This approach was recommended by several experts in tobacco biomarker research [Benowitz 2008; Bernert 2008; Hecht 2008]. In recently published ETS studies, researchers have chosen different approaches regarding creatinine adjustment [Parsons et al. 1998; Trout et al. 1998; Carrer et al. 2000; Anderson et al. 2003; Tulunay et al. 2005; Stark et al. 2007]. Creatinine adjustment can account for potential dilutional effects when measuring biomarkers in spot urine samples. However, according to Barr et al. [2005] and Boeniger et al. [1993], creatinine adjustment of biomarkers in populations that vary by age, sex, and race may yield inaccurate results. Because these factors may have affected our results, we presented both methods. We found that the results, with or without adjustment for creatinine, were similar for NNAL but different for COT.

The GM values that we reported for unadjusted urinary COT are similar to those measured in other indoor environments, such as bars, casinos, and restaurants [Trout et al. 1998; Lindgren et al. 1999; Benowitz and Jacob 2001; Johnsson et al. 2003]. Trout et al. [1998] found a GM preshift level of 23.0 ng/mL and postshift level of 33.3 ng/mL with a significant increase in urinary levels of COT ($p < 0.01$) over the shift.

Health Symptom Questionnaire

NP casino dealers reported higher prevalence of respiratory symptoms than the ETS nonexposed group, but none were statistically significant. The 2006 U.S. Surgeon General's Report on ETS found a suggestive causal relationship between ETS exposure and acute and chronic respiratory symptoms as well as adult-onset asthma [DHHS 2006]. Of the 11 NP casino dealers reporting existing asthma, seven reported exacerbations at work. Although limited studies compare workplace ETS exposure and new-onset asthma, studies have shown an association between exposures to ETS at work and increased risk of asthma and asthma-related symptoms [Greer et al. 1993; Flodin et al. 1995; Blanc et al. 1999, Jaakkola et al. 2003]. Workplace ETS exposure has been shown to contribute more to respiratory symptoms than ETS exposure in the home [Larsson et al. 2003; Dhala et al. 2004]. Two studies among bar workers reported that, when ETS exposure was eliminated from the workplace, improvement in respiratory health, including asthma and asthma-related symptoms, was documented [Eisner et al. 1998, Menzies et al. 2006].

The low participation rate of the NP casino dealers (53%) and the small number of participating administrative and engineering casino employees (n=12) may limit our ability to provide a confident estimate of symptom prevalence among these groups. Because we had no administrative or engineering participants from Caesars Palace, the symptom prevalence does not provide information concerning the administrative and engineering workforce at that casino. However, our findings were comparable to several other studies in which ETS-exposed populations had more respiratory symptoms than those in unexposed groups [White et al. 1991; Eisner et al. 1998; Bates et al. 2002; Wakefield et al. 2003; Fidan 2004; Menzies et al. 2006]. Also, although participation was low among the administrative and engineering employees, health symptom prevalence reported among this group also were comparable to those reported in other ETS unexposed work groups. [White et al. 1991; Nelson et al. 1995; Malkin et al. 1996; Bates et al. 2002; Whelan et al. 2003].

Nonrespiratory symptoms, such as eye irritation, nausea, headache, and dizziness, were included in the health symptom questionnaire based on the health concerns reported by casino dealers. NP casino dealers reported a higher prevalence of nausea, headache, and dizziness than administrative and engineering casino employees did, although these differences were not statistically significant. In addition to eye irritation, past studies have examined the role of nonrespiratory health effects, such as nausea and headache, related to ETS exposure in indoor building environments with conflicting results [Norbäck and Edling 1991; Menzies and Bourbeau 1997; Iribarren et al. 2001].

CONCLUSIONS

NP casino dealers at Bally's, Paris, and Caesars Palace casinos are exposed to ETS in the workplace air, and have absorbed an ETS-specific component into their bodies, as demonstrated by detectable levels of urinary NNAL. The increase in NNAL in the urine of most NP casino dealers at the end of their work shift demonstrates that NP casino dealers are exposed to a known carcinogen in the tobacco smoke at the casinos. NP casino dealers reported a higher prevalence of respiratory symptoms than to unexposed workers, but the results were not statistically significant. The best means of eliminating workplace exposure to ETS is to ban all smoking in the casinos.

RECOMMENDATIONS

We recommend eliminating tobacco from the casinos and implementing a smoking cessation program. The casinos should also eliminate smoking near building entrances and air intakes to protect employees from involuntary exposure to ETS. A physician should evaluate employees with respiratory symptoms, especially symptoms related to asthma that are associated with workplace exposures.

We recommend that if any modifications are made to the ventilation systems, they should be done in adherence with current ASHRAE-recommended guidelines [ANSI/ASHRAE 2007]. In addition, a preventive maintenance plan should be developed for the ventilation systems. This should include testing and balancing the systems and regular calibration of the CO_2 sensors in the return air ducts.

We also recommend better communication between employees and management about occupational health and safety issues. One way to achieve this would be for employee and management representatives to form joint health and safety committees to address workplace health and safety concerns. These committees should meet regularly and be given needed resources to address ongoing health and safety issues.

REFERENCES

Anderson KE, Kliris J, Murphy L, Carmella SG, Han S, Link C, Bliss RL, Puumala S, Murphy SE, Hecht SS [2003]. Metabolites of a tobacco-specific lung carcinogen in nonsmoking casino patrons. Cancer Epidemiol Biomarkers Prev 12(12):1544–1546.

ANSI/ASHRAE [2004]. Thermal environmental conditions for human occupancy, standard 55-2004: thermal environmental conditions for human occupancy. Atlanta, GA: American Society of Heating, Refrigerating, and Air-Conditioning Engineers, Inc.

ANSI/ASHRAE [2007]. Ventilation for acceptable indoor air quality, standard 62-2007. Atlanta, GA: American Society of Heating, Refrigerating, and Air-Conditioning Engineers, Inc.

ASHRAE [2005]. Environmental tobacco smoke. Position document. Atlanta, GA: American Society of Heating, Refrigerating and Air-Conditioning Engineers, Inc.

Barr DB, Wilder LC, Caudill SP, Gonzalez AJ, Needham LL, Pirkle JL [2005]. Urinary creatinine concentrations in the U.S. population: implications for urinary biologic monitoring measurements. Environ Health Perspect 113(2):192–200.

Bates MN, Fawcett J, Dickson S, Berezowski R, Garrett N [2002]. Exposure of hospitality workers to environmental tobacco smoke. Tob Control 11(2):125–129.

Benowitz NL [1999]. Biomarkers of environmental tobacco smoke exposure. Environ Health Perspect 107(2)(Suppl):349s–355s.

Benowitz NL, Jacob P [2001]. Trans-3'-hydroxyCOT: disposition kinetics, effects, and plasma levels during cigarette smoking. Br J Clin Pharmacol 51(1):53–59.

Benowitz NL (nbenowitz@medsfgh.ucsf.edu) [2008]. Request for assistance on ETS biomarkers. Private email message to Christine West (cawest@cdc.gov), May 23.

Bernert JT (Jbernert@cdc.gov) [2008]. Request for assistance on ETS biomarkers. Private email message to Christine West (cawest@cdc.gov), May 23.

Blanc PD, Ellbjar S, Jandon C, Norback D, Norrman E, Plaschke P, Toren K [1999]. Asthma-related work disability in Sweden. The impact of workplace exposures. Am J Respir Crit Care Med 160(3):2028–2033.

Boeniger MF, Lowry LK, Rosenberg J [1993]. Interpretation of urine results used to assess chemical exposure with emphasis on creatinine adjustments: a review. Am Ind Hyg Assoc J 54(10):615–627.

Burnett RT, Dales RE, Raizenne ME, Krewski D, Summers PW, Roberts GR, Raad-Young M, Dann T, Brook J [1994]. Effects of low ambient levels of ozone and sulfates on the frequency of respiratory admissions to Ontario hospitals. Environ Res 65(2):172–194.

Carrer P, Maroni M, Alcinin D, Cavallo D, Fustinoni S, Lovato L, Visigalli F [2000]. Assessment through environmental and biological measurements of total daily exposure to volatile organic compounds of office workers in Milan, Italy. Indoor Air 10(4):258–268.

Dhala A, Pinsker K, Prezant DJ [2004]. Respiratory health consequences of environmental tobacco smoke. Med Clin North Am 88(6):1535–1552.

DHHS [2006]. The health consequences of involuntary exposure to tobacco smoke: A report of the Surgeon General. Washington, DC: U.S. Government Printing Office, Washington, DC.

Eisner MD, Smith AK, Blanc PD [1998]. Bartenders' respiratory health after establishment of smoke-free bars and taverns. JAMA 280(22):1909–1914.

EPA [2008]. Naphthalene. [www.epa.gov/ttn/atw/hlthef/naphthal.html]. Date accessed: January 15, 2009.

Fidan F, Cimrin AH, Ergor G, Sevinc C [2004]. Airway disease risk from environmental tobacco smoke among coffeehouse workers in Turkey. Tob Control 13(2):161–166.

Flodin U, Jeonsson P, Ziegler J, Axelson O [1995]. An epidemiologic study of bronchial asthma and smoking. Epidemiology 6(5):503–505.

REFERENCES
(CONTINUED)

Greer JR, Abbey DE, Burchette RJ [1993]. Asthma related to occupational and ambient air pollutants in nonsmokers. J Occup Med 35(9):909–915.

Grimmer G, Naujack KW [1987]. Gas chromatographic determination of polycyclic aromatic hydrocarbons in sidestream and mainstreanm smoke and the air of enclosed environments. In: O'Neill IK, Bruenemann KD, Dodet B, Hoffmann D, eds. Environmental carcinogenesis-methods of analysis and exposure assessments, volume 9-passive smoking. IARC Scientific Publications No. 810, International Agency for Research on Cancer, Lyon, pp. 249–268.

Hecht SS, Carmella SG, Chen M, Dor Koch JF, Miller AT, Murphy SE, Jensen JA, Zimmerman CL, Hatsukami DK [1999]. Quantitation of urinary metabolites of a tobacco-specific lung carcinogen after smoking cessation. Cancer Res 59(3):590–596.

Hecht SS [2002]. Human urinary carcinogen metabolites: biomarkers for investigating tobacco and cancer. Carcinogenesis 23(6):907–922.

Hecht SS (hecht002@umn.edu) [2008]. Request for assistance on ETS biomarkers. Private email message to Christine West (cawest@cdc.gov), May 23.

Hornung RW, Reed LD [1990]. Estimation of average concentration in the presence of non-detectable values. Appl Occup Environ Hyg 5(1):46–51.

Husgafvel-Pursiainen K, Sorsa M, Moller M, Benestad C [1986]. Genotoxicity and polynuclear aromatic hydrocarbon analysis of environmental tobacco smoke samples from restaurants Mutagenesis 1(4):287–292.

Iribarren C, Friedman GD, Klatsky AL, Eisner MD [2001]. Exposure to environmental tobacco smoke: association with personal characteristics and self reported health conditions. J Epidemiol Community Health 55(10):721–728.

Jaakkola MS, Piipari R, Jaakkola N, Jaakkola JJ [2003]. Environmental tobacco smoke and adult-onset asthma: a population-based incident case-control study. Am J Public Health 93(12):2055–2060.

REFERENCES
(CONTINUED)

Jenkins RA, Counts RW [1999]. Occupational exposure to environmental tobacco smoke, results of two personal exposure studies. Environ Health Perspec 107(Suppl 2):341–348.

Johnsson T, Tuomi T, Hyvarinen M, Svinhufvud J, Rothberg M, Reijula K [2003]. Occupational exposure of non-smoking restaurant personnel to environmental tobacco smoke in Finland. Am J Ind Med 43(5):523–531.

Larsson ML, Loit HM, Meren M, Polluste J, Magnusson A, Larsson K, Lundback B [2003]. Passive smoking and respiratory symptoms in the FinEsS Study. Eur Respir J 21(4):672–676.

Lindgren T, Willers S, Skarping G, Norbäck D [1999]. Urinary COT concentration in flight attendants, in relation to exposure to environmental tobacco smoke during intercontinental flights. Int Arch Occup Environ Health 72(7):475–479.

Lippy BE, Turner RW [1991]. Complex mixtures in industrial workspaces: lessons for indoor air quality evaluations. Environ Health Perspect 95:81–83.

Malkin R, Wilcox R, Sieber K [1996]. The National Institute for Occupational Safety and Health indoor environmental evaluation experience. Part two: Symptom prevalence. Appl Occup Environ Hyg 11(6):540–545.

Menzies D, Bourbeau J [1997]. Building-related illnesses. New Eng J Med 337(21):1524–1531.

Menzies D, Nair A, Williamson PA, Schembri S, Al-Khairalla MZH, Barnes M, Fardon TC, McFarlane L, Magee GJ, Lipworth BJ [2006]. Respiratory symptoms, pulmonary function and markers of inflammation among bar workers before and after a legislative ban on smoking in public places. JAMA 296(14):1742–1748.

Nelson NA, Kaufman JD, Burt J, Karr C [1995]. Health symptoms and the work environment in four nonproblem office buildings. Scand J Work Environ Health 21(1):51–59.

Norbäck D, Edling C [1991]. Environmental, occupational, and personal factors related to the prevalence of sick building syndrome in the general population. Br J Ind Med 48(7):451–462.

Ogden MW, Maiolo KC [1989]. Collection and determination of solanesol as a tracer of environmental tobacco smoke in indoor air. Environ Sci Technol 23(9):1148–1154.

Parsons WD, Carmella SG, Akerkar S, Bonilla LE, Hecht SS [1998]. A metabolite of the tobacco-specific lung carcinogen 4-(methylnitrosamino)-1-(3-pyridyl)-1-butanone in the urine of hospital workers exposed to environmental tobacco smoke. Cancer Epid Biomarkers Prev 7(3):257–260.

Phillips K, Howard DA, Bentley M, Alvan G [1998]. Measured exposures by personal monitoring for respirable suspended particles and environmental tobacco smoke of housewives and office workers resident in Bremen, Germany. Int Arch Occup Environ Health 71(3):201–212.

Pope CA [2000]. Epidemiology of fine particulate air pollution and human health: biologic mechanisms and who's at risk? Environ Health Perspect 108(Suppl 4):713–723.

Pirkle JL, Flegal KM, Bernert JT, Brody DJ, Etzel RA, Maurer KR [1996]. Exposure of the U.S. population to environmental tobacco smoke. The third national health and nutrition examination survey, 1988 to 1991. JAMA 275(16):1233–1240.

Sheppard L, Levy D, Norris G, Larson TV, Koenig JQ [1999]. Effects of ambient air pollution on nonelderly asthma hospital admissions in Seattle, Washington, 1987–1994. Epidemiology 10(1):23–30.

Stark MJ, Rohde K, Maher JE, Pizacani BA, Dent CW, Bard R, Carmella SG, Benoit AR, Thomson NM, Hecht SS [2007]. The impact of clean indoor air exemptions and preemption policies on the prevalence of a tobacco-specific lung carcinogen among nonsmoking bar and restaurant workers. Am J Public Health 97(8):1457–1463.

Tang H, Richards G, Benner CL, Tuominen JP, Lee ML, Lewis EA, Hansen LD, Eatough DJ [1990]. Solanesol: a tracer for environmental tobacco smoke particles. Environ Sci Technol 24(6):848–852.

Trout D, Decker J, Mueller C, Bernert JT, Pirkle J [1998]. Exposure of casino employees to environmental tobacco smoke. J Occup Environ Med 40(3):270–276.

REFERENCES
(CONTINUED)

Tucker SP, Pretty JR [2005]. Identification of oxidation products of solanesol produced during air sampling for tobacco smoke by electrospray mass spectrometry and HPLC. Analyst *130*(10):1414–1424.

Tulunay OE, Hecht SS, Carmella SG, Zhang Y, Lemmonds C, Murphy S, Hatsukami DK [2005]. Urinary metabolites of a tobacco-specific lung carcinogen in nonsmoking hospitality workers. Cancer Epidemiol Biomarkers Prev *14*(5):1283–1286.

Wakefield M, Trotter L, Cameron M, Woodward A, Inglis G, Hill D [2003]. Association between exposure to workplace secondhand smoke and reported respiratory and sensory symptoms: cross-sectional study. J Occup Environ Med *45*(6):622–627.

Whelan EA, Lawson CC, Grajewski B, Peterson MR, Pinkerton LE, Ward EM, Schnorr TM [2003]. Prevalence of respiratory symptoms among female flight attendants and teachers. J Occup Environ Med *60*(12):929–934.

White JR, Froeb HF, Kulik JA [1991]. Respiratory illness in nonsmokers chronically exposed to tobacco smoke in the workplace. Chest *100*(1):39–43.

Employee Interviews (July 2005)

During private medical interviews and in open discussions, employees reported a range of health symptoms and conditions they believed were related to exposure to ETS during their work in the casino. These included four types of cancer (types not reported here for reasons of confidentiality), respiratory symptoms and illnesses (asthma, emphysema), mucous membrane irritation, dizziness, nausea, headaches, and cardiovascular problems, such as heart attacks and strokes.

Summary of OSHA Logs

Bally's and Paris Casinos

No respiratory-related symptoms or illnesses were recorded for Bally's or Paris casino dealers in 2003, 2004, or 2005.

Caesars Palace Casino

No respiratory symptoms or illnesses were recorded for Caesars Palace casino dealers in 1999, 2000, 2001, and 2003. Two Caesars Palace casino dealers reported eye irritation in 2000 and 2001, and one dealer reported "disease of respiratory system" in 2004. None of these resulted in any lost work days. OSHA Logs were not available for 2002 and 2005 from Caesars Palace.

APPENDIX B: VENTILATION OVERVIEW

Bally's Casino

The HVAC system originally began operating in 1974 and was updated in 1981. Bally's HVAC filtration design was reported as a single bank of pleated filters with an estimated filtration efficiency rating of MERV 8 [ANSI/ASHRAE 1999]. We discussed the design and retrofit of Bally's HVAC system with the ventilation engineer. This engineer described Bally's as an older facility that has many generations of HVAC equipment serving the gaming area. He estimated that outdoor air set points and equipment selection were likely determined using the 1973 and 1981 editions of ASHRAE Standard 62 [ASHRAE 1973, 1981]. The actual supply rates of outdoor air delivered to the occupied zones were not evaluated by NIOSH and were unknown.

Paris Casino

The current HVAC system, designed by JBA Consulting Engineers (Las Vegas, Nevada), began operating in 1999. According to the ventilation engineers, several factors govern the outdoor air delivery for Paris:

1. The building is designed with variable air volume HVAC systems that are intended to maintain the building at a positive pressure.

2. The maximum amount of outdoor air designated for normal operation of each air handler is determined by its cooling capacity and the outdoor design temperatures.

3. Minimum outdoor air set points are established for each air handler to meet the JBA engineer's outdoor air supply objectives. Based on conversations with JBA's engineer, the Paris set points would have been selected using the Ventilation Rate Table procedure specified in the 1989 edition of ASHRAE Standard 62, *Ventilation for Acceptable Indoor Air Quality* [ANSI/ASHRAE 1989]. This procedure prescribes the minimum supply rate of outdoor air (30 cfm/person) based upon the number of people and an assumed population density within the gaming areas. The actual supply rate of outdoor air delivered to the occupied zone at these supply rates was not evaluated by NIOSH and was unknown.

4. The Paris HVAC system monitors concentrations of CO_2 in the return air ducts. If the CO_2 concentration exceeds 800 ppm, the HVAC system reportedly switches to 100% outdoor air supply.

5. The Paris HVAC systems use an economizer cycle based on the outdoor dry bulb temperature. Whenever this temperature falls below 72°F, the economizer switches to 100% outdoor air supply. The ventilation engineers estimated this condition occurs approximately 8 months of the year.

6. The Paris HVAC filtration systems were reported to be two-bank systems comprised of a 2" pleated prefilter followed by a bag filter with an estimated 80%–95% dust spot efficiency [ANSI/ASHRAE 1992].

Caesars Palace Casino

The HVAC system was renovated in 1996 with the design assistance of JBA Consulting Engineers (Las Vegas, Nevada). The following HVAC concept of operation was reported by the Caesars Palace facility engineering representatives:

1. The building is designed with variable air volume HVAC systems that are intended to maintain the building at a positive pressure.

2. The minimum outdoor air set point is 40%. The actual supply rate of outdoor air delivered to the occupied zone at this set point was not evaluated by NIOSH and was unknown. However, in subsequent telephone conversations with JBA's engineer, we learned that the Caesars Palace outdoor air supply rates would have been selected using the Ventilation Rate Table procedure specified in the 1989 edition of ASHRAE Standard 62 for the newer (1996) equipment. Older HVAC equipment could be up to 30 years old and would use different outdoor air supply rates based upon the applicable version of ASHRAE Standard 62 in effect at that time.

3. The Caesars Palace HVAC system also monitors concentrations of CO_2 in the return air ducts. If the CO_2 levels exceed 600 ppm, the HVAC system is designed to switch to 100% outdoor air supply. The Caesars Palace representatives did not know when the last time this monitor had been calibrated, replaced, or otherwise maintained. The engineer stated that these are generally solid-state units that require replacement approximately every 2 years.

4. The Caesars Palace HVAC system uses an economizer cycle based on the outdoor temperature. Whenever this temperature falls below 68°F, the economizer switches to 100% outdoor air supply. The Caesars Palace engineers estimated that this condition occurs 4 months of the year.

5. The Caesars Palace HVAC filtration system was described as a single-bank pleated filter with a MERV 8 filtration efficiency rating.

References

ASHRAE [1973]. Standards for natural and mechanical ventilation, standard 62. Atlanta, GA: American Society of Heating, Refrigerating, and Air-Conditioning Engineers, Inc.

ASHRAE [1981]. Ventilation for acceptable indoor air quality, standard 62. Atlanta, GA: American Society of Heating, Refrigerating, and Air-Conditioning Engineers, Inc.

ANSI/ASHRAE [1989]. Ventilation for acceptable indoor air quality, standard 62. Atlanta, GA: American Society of Heating, Refrigerating, and Air-Conditioning Engineers, Inc.

ANSI/ASHRAE [1992]. Gravimetric and dust-spot procedures for testing air-cleaning devices used in general ventilation for removing particulate matter standard 52.1. Atlanta, GA: American Society of Heating, Refrigerating, and Air-Conditioning Engineers, Inc.

ANSI/ASHRAE [1999]. Method of testing general ventilation air-cleaning devices for removal efficiency by particle size, standard 52.2. Atlanta, GA: American Society of Heating, Refrigerating, and Air-Conditioning Engineers, Inc.

Cotinine

Urinary COT was analyzed using a solid-phase competitive chemiluminescent immunoassay. Beads coated with polyclonal rabbit anti-COT antibody, 20 μL of sample, and alkaline phosphatase conjugated COT were incubated for 30 minutes. The beads were then washed, and chemiluminescent substrate was added. Detection of COT is reflected by the amount of light output measured by a photometer. The assay LOD was 5 ng/mL, and the LOQ was 10 ng/mL. Assay adjustors and controls were used as recommended by the manufacturer.

4-(Methylnitrosamino)-1-(3-Pyridyl)-1-Butanol and Creatinine

Analysis of total NNAL in urine samples was performed by using an HPLC/API-MS combined with a novel sample clean-up using solid-phase extraction based on a molecularly imprinted polymer column developed specifically for this assay. Urine creatinine levels were measured enzymatically by the Roche CREA Plus procedure using a Hitachi analyzer [Xia et al. 2005]. The LOD for this analysis is 0.0030 ng/mL (3 pg/mL).

Nicotine and 4-Vinyl Pyridine

NIC and 4-VP were simultaneously sampled and analyzed per NIOSH Method 2551 [NIOSH 2008]. NIC was collected on XAD-4™ tubes at a flow rate of 1.5 Lpm and analyzed using a GC equipped with a nitrogen phosphorous detector.

Polynuclear Aromatic Hydrocarbons

The particulate and vapor phases of PAHs were sampled simultaneously using glass fiber filters for the particulate phase and OVS tubes with XAD-7™ sorbent for the vapor phase. Samples were collected at a flow rate of 2.0 Lpm and analyzed for 16 individual PAHs using a GC equipped with a flame ionization detector. The sampling and analysis method for PAHs is a modification of NIOSH Method 5515 [NIOSH 2008].

Respirable Suspended Particulates

RSP was sampled and gravimetrically analyzed per a modification of NIOSH Method 0600 [NIOSH 2008]. Samples were collected using a BGI4L cyclone (BGI Incorporated, Waltham, Massachusetts) on 37-mm, 1.0 μm pore size, PTFE filters housed in black, opaque polypropylene 3-piece cassettes at a flow rate of 2.2 Lpm.

Appendix C: Methodology
(continued)

Solanesol

SOL was extracted from the RSP PTFE filters using methanol and analyzed using an HPLC equipped with a UV detector according to a modification of ASTM method D-6271-04. The ASTM method was modified to use a C 8 column for HPLC separation and analysis [ASTM 2004].

Volatile Organic Compounds

VOCs were collected on charcoal tubes at a flow rate of 100 mL/min and analyzed per NIOSH Method 2501 [NIOSH 2008].

Aldehydes

FLD and ACTLD air samples were collected on passive badges (UMEX™, SKC Inc., Eighty-Four, Pennsylvania) impregnated with 2,4-dinitrophenylhydrazine, and analyzed using an HPLC per NIOSH Method 2016 [NIOSH 2008].

Carbon Monoxide

Area samples for CO were collected using a QTRAK Plus® (TSI, St. Paul, Minnesota) equipped with an electrochemical sensor. Data was logged at one-minute intervals and downloaded onto a laptop computer. The instruments were calibrated daily using calibration gas.

References

ASTM [2004]. ASTM D6271 - 04 Standard test method for estimating contribution of environmental tobacco smoke to respirable suspended particles based on solanesol. ASTM International, 100 Barr Harbor Drive, PO Box C700, West Conshohocken, PA, 19428-2959 USA.

NIOSH [2008]. NIOSH manual of analytical methods (NMAM®). 4th ed. Schlecht PC, O'Connor PF, eds. Cincinnati, OH: U.S. Department of Health and Human Services, Centers for Disease Control and Prevention, National Institute for Occupational Safety and Health, DHHS (NIOSH) Publication 94-113 (August, 1994); 1st Supplement Publication 96-135, 2nd Supplement Publication 98-119; 3rd Supplement 2003-154. [www.cdc.gov/niosh/nmam/].

Xia Y, McGuffey JE, Bhattacharyya S, Sellergren B, Yilmaz E, Wang L, Bernert JT [2005]. Analysis of the tobacco-specific nitrosamine 4-(methylnitrosamino)-1-(3-pyridyl)-1-butanol in urine by extraction on a molecularly imprinted polymer column and liquid chromatography/atmospheric pressure ionization tandem mass spectrometry. Anal Chem 77(23):7639–7645.

APPENDIX D: OCCUPATIONAL EXPOSURE LIMITS & HEALTH EFFECTS

In evaluating the hazards posed by workplace exposures, NIOSH investigators use both mandatory (legally enforceable) and recommended OELs for chemical, physical, and biological agents as a guide for making recommendations. OELs have been developed by Federal agencies and safety and health organizations to prevent the occurrence of adverse health effects from workplace exposures. Generally, OELs suggest levels of exposure to which most workers may be exposed up to 10 hours per day, 40 hours per week for a working lifetime without experiencing adverse health effects. However, not all workers will be protected from adverse health effects even if their exposures are maintained below these levels. A small percentage may experience adverse health effects because of individual susceptibility, a pre-existing medical condition, and/or a hypersensitivity (allergy). In addition, some hazardous substances may act in combination with other workplace exposures, the general environment, or with medications or personal habits of the worker to produce health effects even if the occupational exposures are controlled at the level set by the exposure limit. Also, some substances can be absorbed by direct contact with the skin and mucous membranes in addition to being inhaled, which contributes to the individual's overall exposure.

Most OELs are expressed as a TWA exposure. A TWA refers to the average exposure during a normal 8- to 10-hour workday. Some chemical substances and physical agents have recommended STEL or ceiling values where health effects are caused by exposures over a short period. Unless otherwise noted, the STEL is a 15-minute TWA exposure that should not be exceeded at any time during a workday, and the ceiling limit is an exposure that should not be exceeded at any time.

In the United States, OELs have been established by Federal agencies, professional organizations, state and local governments, and other entities. Some OELs are legally enforceable limits, while others are recommendations. The U.S. Department of Labor OSHA PELs (29 CFR 1910 [general industry]; 29 CFR 1926 [construction industry]; and 29 CFR 1917 [maritime industry]) are legal limits enforceable in workplaces covered under the Occupational Safety and Health Act. NIOSH RELs are recommendations based on a critical review of the scientific and technical information available on a given hazard and the adequacy of methods to identify and control the hazard. NIOSH RELs can be found in the *NIOSH Pocket Guide to Chemical Hazards* [NIOSH 2005]. NIOSH also recommends different types of risk management practices (e.g., engineering controls, safe work practices, worker education/training, personal protective equipment, and exposure and medical monitoring) to minimize the risk of exposure and adverse health effects from these hazards. Other OELs that are commonly used and cited in the United States include the TLVs recommended by ACGIH, a professional organization, and the WEELs recommended by the American Industrial Hygiene Association, another professional organization. The TLVs and WEELs are developed by committee members of these associations from a review of the published, peer-reviewed literature. They are not consensus standards. ACGIH TLVs are considered voluntary exposure guidelines for use by industrial hygienists and others trained in this discipline "to assist in the control of health hazards" [ACGIH 2007]. WEELs have been established for some chemicals "when no other legal or authoritative limits exist" [AIHA 2007].

Outside the United States, OELs have been established by various agencies and organizations and include both legal and recommended limits. Since 2006, the Berufsgenossenschaftliches Institut für Arbeitsschutz (German Institute for Occupational Safety and Health) has maintained a database of international OELs from European Union member states, Canada (Québec), Japan, Switzerland, and the United States available at www.hvbg.de/e/bia/gestis/limit_values/index.html. The database contains international limits for over 1250 hazardous substances and is updated annually.

Employers should understand that not all hazardous chemicals have specific OSHA PELs, and for some agents the legally enforceable and recommended limits may not reflect current health-based information. However, an employer is still required by OSHA to protect its employees from hazards even in the absence of a specific OSHA PEL. OSHA requires an employer to furnish employees a place of employment free from recognized hazards that cause or are likely to cause death or serious physical harm [Occupational Safety and Health Act of 1970 (Public Law 91–596, sec. 5(a)(1))]. Thus, NIOSH investigators encourage employers to make use of other OELs when making risk assessment and risk management decisions to best protect the health of their employees. NIOSH investigators also encourage the use of the traditional hierarchy of controls approach to eliminate or minimize identified workplace hazards. This includes, in order of preference, the use of: (1) substitution or elimination of the hazardous agent, (2) engineering controls (e.g., local exhaust ventilation, process enclosure, dilution ventilation), (3) administrative controls (e.g., limiting time of exposure, employee training, work practice changes, medical surveillance), and (4) personal protective equipment (e.g., respiratory protection, gloves, eye protection, hearing protection). Control banding, a qualitative risk assessment and risk management tool, is a complementary approach to protecting worker health that focuses resources on exposure controls by describing how a risk needs to be managed. Information regarding control banding is available at www.cdc.gov/niosh/topics/ctrlbanding/. This approach can be applied in situations where OELs have not been established or can be used to supplement the OELs, when available.

Environmental Tobacco Smoke

Exposure criteria for ETS have not been established, although NIOSH and others have determined that ETS is associated with an increased risk of lung cancer, other lung disease, and possibly heart disease. More than 4,000 compounds have been identified in ETS, many of which exert their biologic properties through different mechanisms. A common strategy for assessing exposure to ETS is to monitor one or more "marker" substances and use these as an index of exposure. Selection of these compounds is based on their ease of measurement and specificity to ETS, and not necessarily because they are the most toxic components of ETS.

In this survey, vapor-phase NIC, RSP, VOCs, PAHs, and ALD were monitored as marker substances. The concentrations of these markers in ETS are consistently lower than their respective OELs, which are based primarily on acute effects. The NIOSH REL and the ACGIH TLV for NIC, used in the agricultural industry, are 500 µg/m³ [NIOSH 1992; ACGIH 2007]. OSHA has no corresponding PEL. In contrast, the mean area air NIC concentrations reported in ETS studies of public buildings have ranged from 0.7–37 µg/m³; concentrations in restaurants and bars have ranged from 2.3–65.5 µg/m³; and concentrations in gaming parlors and betting shops have ranged from 11–19 µg/m³. Full-shift respirable particulate measurements using gravimetric analysis have ranged up to 80 µg/m³ in office buildings [Miesner et al.

1998] and up to 253 µg/m^3 in restaurants [Brauer and Mannetje 1989]. The NIOSH and OSHA criteria for NIC and RSP are not applicable to ETS exposures, particularly because these contaminants are measured only as markers of ETS exposure [NIOSH 2005; 29 CFR 1910].

Temperature and Relative Humidity

Temperature and RH measurements are often collected as part of an IEQ investigation because these parameters affect the perception of comfort in an indoor environment. The perception of thermal comfort is related to an individual's metabolic heat production, the transfer of heat to the environment, physiological adjustments, and body temperature [NIOSH 1986]. Heat transfer from the body to the environment is influenced by factors such as temperature, humidity, air movement, personal activities, and clothing. The ANSI/ASHRAE Standard 55-2004, *Thermal Environmental Conditions for Human Occupancy*, specifies conditions in which 80% or more of the occupants would be expected to find the environment thermally acceptable [ANSI/ASHRAE 2004]. Assuming slow air movement (under 40 fpm) and 50% RH, the operative temperatures recommended by ASHRAE range from 68 5°F to 76°F in the winter, and from 75°F to 80.5°F in the summer. The difference between the two is largely due to seasonal clothing selection. ASHRAE also recommends maintaining RH at or below 65% [ANSI/ASHRAE 2007]. Excessive humidity can promote the excessive growth of microorganisms and dust mites.

Carbon Dioxide

CO_2 is a normal constituent of exhaled breath and is not considered a building air pollutant. It can be used as an indicator of whether sufficient quantities of outdoor air are being introduced into an occupied space for acceptable odor control. However, CO_2 is not an effective indicator of ventilation adequacy if the ventilated area is not occupied at its usual occupant density at the time the CO_2 is measured. ASHRAE notes in an informative appendix to standard 62.1 that indoor CO_2 concentrations no greater than 700 ppm above outdoor CO_2 concentrations will satisfy a substantial majority (about 80%) of visitors with regard to odor from sedentary building occupants (body odor) [ANSI/ASHRAE 2007]. Elevated CO_2 concentrations suggest that other indoor contaminants may also be increased. If CO_2 concentrations are elevated, the amount of outdoor air introduced into the ventilated space may need to be increased. When CO_2 concentrations are used as an indicator to determine outdoor air requirements, ventilation system designs that rely on duct-mounted CO_2 sensors should have some form of ventilation efficiency documentation that relates concentration values observed at the duct location with those observed within the breathing zone of the occupied space.

Carbon Monoxide

CO is a colorless, odorless, tasteless gas that can be a product of the incomplete combustion of organic compounds. CO combines with hemoglobin and interferes with the oxygen-carrying capacity of blood.

Symptoms include headache, drowsiness, dizziness, nausea, vomiting, collapse, myocardial ischemia, and death [Hathaway et al. 1991]. The NIOSH REL for CO is 35 ppm for up to a 10-hour TWA. NIOSH also recommends a ceiling limit of 200 ppm, which should not be exceeded at any time during the workday. The ACGIH TLV for an 8-hour TWA is 25 ppm; the OSHA PEL for an 8-hour TWA is 50 ppm.

References

ACGIH® [2007]. 2007 TLVs® and BEIs®: threshold limit values for chemical substances and physical agents. Cincinnati, OH: American Conference of Governmental Industrial Hygienists.

AIHA [2007]. 2007 Emergency response planning guidelines (ERPG) & workplace environmental exposure levels (WEEL) handbook. Fairfax, VA: American Industrial Hygiene Association.

ANSI/ASHRAE [2004]. Thermal environmental conditions for human occupancy, standard 55-2004. Atlanta, GA: American Society for Heating, Refrigerating, and Air-Conditioning Engineers, Inc.

ANSI/ASHRAE [2007]. Ventilation for acceptable indoor air quality, standard 62.1-2007. Atlanta, GA: American Society of Heating, Refrigerating, and Air-Conditioning Engineers, Inc.

Brauer M, Mannetje A [1998]. Restaurant smoking restrictions and environmental tobacco smoke exposure. Am J Public Health 88(12):1834–1836.

CFR. Code of Federal Regulations. Washington, DC: U.S. Government Printing Office, Office of the Federal Register.

Hathaway GJ, Proctor NH, Hughes JP, Fischman ML [1991]. Chemical hazards of the workplace. 3rd ed. New York, NY: Van Nostrand Reinhold.

Miesner EA, Rudnick SN, Hu FC, Spengler JD, Preller L, Özkaynak H, Nelson W [1989]. Particulate and nicotine sampling in public facilities and offices. JAPCA 39(12):1577–1582.

NIOSH [1986]. Criteria for a recommended standard: occupational exposure to hot environments, revised criteria. Cincinnati, OH: U.S. Department of Health and Human Services, Centers for Disease Control, National Institute for Occupational Safety and Health, DHHS (NIOSH) Publication No. 86-13.

NIOSH [1992]. Recommendations for occupational safety and health: compendium of policy documents and statements. Cincinnati, OH: U.S. Department of Health and Human Services, Centers for Disease Control and Prevention, National Institute for Occupational Safety and Health, DHHS (NIOSH) Publication No. 92-100.

NIOSH [2005]. NIOSH pocket guide to chemical hazards. Cincinnati, OH: U.S. Department of Health and Human Services, Centers for Disease Control and Prevention, National Institute for Occupational Safety and Health, DHHS (NIOSH) Publication No. 2005-149. [www.cdc.gov/niosh/npg/]. Date accessed: January 15, 2009.

The Hazard Evaluations and Technical Assistance Branch (HETAB) of the National Institute for Occupational Safety and Health (NIOSH) conducts field investigations of possible health hazards in the workplace. These investigations are conducted under the authority of Section 20(a)(6) of the Occupational Safety and Health (OSHA) Act of 1970, 29 U.S.C. 669(a)(6), which authorizes the Secretary of Health and Human Services, following a written request from any employer or authorized representative of employees, to determine whether any substance normally found in the place of employment has potentially toxic effects in such concentrations as used or found. HETAB also provides, upon request, technical and consultative assistance to federal, state, and local agencies; labor; industry; and other groups or individuals to control occupational health hazards and to prevent related trauma and disease.

The findings and conclusions in this report are those of the authors and do not necessarily represent the views of NIOSH. Mention of any company or product does not constitute endorsement by NIOSH. In addition, citations to websites external to NIOSH do not constitute NIOSH endorsement of the sponsoring organizations or their programs or products. Furthermore, NIOSH is not responsible for the content of these websites. All Web addresses referenced in this document were accessible as of the publication date.

This report was prepared by Chandran Achutan, Christine West, Charles Mueller, and Yvonne Boudreau of HETAB, Division of Surveillance, Hazard Evaluations and Field Studies (DSHEFS), and Kenneth Mead of the Engineering and Physical Hazards Branch, Division of Applied Research and Technology (DART). Field assistance was provided by Ayodele Adebayo, Donnie Booher, Greg Burr, Lisa Delaney, Judith Eisenberg, Lynda Ewers, Brad King, Manny Rodriguez, Dave Sylvain, Sangwoo Tak, and Loren Tapp of HETAB; Kevin L. Dunn from the Industrywide Studies Branch in DSHEFS; Stewart Curtis from Loma Linda University; and Shirley Robertson and Debbie Sammons from the Biomonitoring and Health Assessment Branch, DART. Analytical support was provided by Tom Bernert and Charles Dodson in the Tobacco Exposure Biomarkers Section of the National Center for Environmental Health (Atlanta, Georgia), DataChem Laboratories (Salt Lake City, Utah), and by Ardith Grote of DART.

ACKNOWLEDGMENTS AND AVAILABILITY OF REPORT
(CONTINUED)

Health communication assistance was provided by Stefanie Evans. Editorial assistance was provided by Ellen Galloway. Desktop publishing was performed by Robin Smith.

Copies of this report have been sent to employee and management representatives at Bally's, Paris, and Caesars Palace Casinos in Las Vegas, Nevada; and the OSHA Regional Office. This report is not copyrighted and may be freely reproduced. The report may be viewed and printed at www.cdc.gov/niosh/hhe. Copies may be purchased from the National Technical Information Service at 5825 Port Royal Road, Springfield, Virginia 22161.